50/61

17.95

Everything You Need to Know About

Lyme Disease

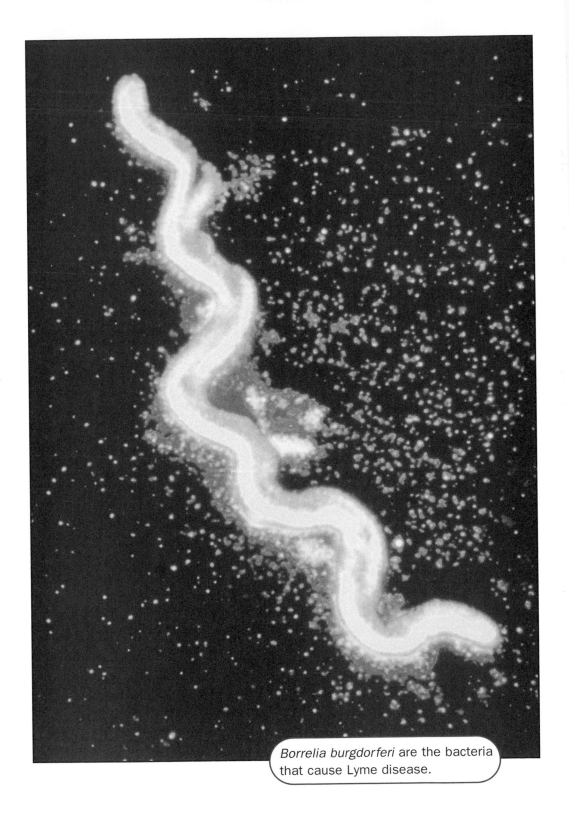

Borrelia burgdorferi are the bacteria that cause Lyme disease.

Everything You Need to Know About

Lyme Disease

Karen Donnelly

The Rosen Publishing Group, Inc.
New York

As always, this book is dedicated to my husband, David, and my beautiful and brilliant daughters, Cathy and Colleen. This book, though, is especially dedicated to Colleen who, when she was seven years old, suffered through the arthritis symptoms of Lyme disease.

Published in 2000 by The Rosen Publishing Group, Inc.
29 East 21st Street, New York, NY 10010

Copyright © 2000 by The Rosen Publishing Group, Inc.

First Edition

Library of Congress Cataloging-in-Publication Data

Donnelly, Karen
     Everything you need to know about Lyme disease / Karen Donnelly.
         p. cm. — (The need to know library)
     Includes bibliographical references and index.
     Summary: Describes the causes, symptoms, and treatment of Lyme disease.
     ISBN 0-8239-3216-8
     1. Lyme disease—Juvenile literature. [1. Lyme disease 2. Diseases.] I. Title. II. Series.

RC155.5.D66 2000
616.9'2 —dc21
                                                                    99-086258

Manufactured in the United States of America

Contents

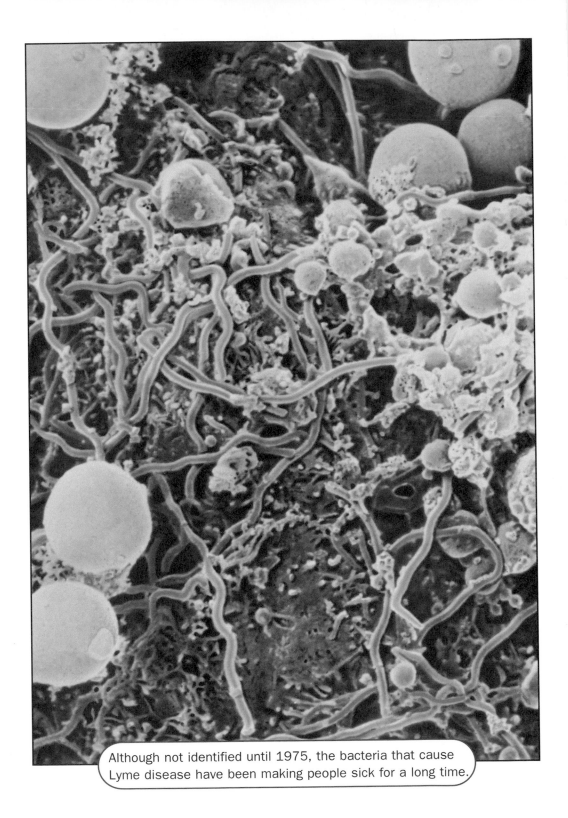

Although not identified until 1975, the bacteria that cause Lyme disease have been making people sick for a long time.

Chapter One

What Is Lyme Disease?

Some people believe Lyme disease is a new disease. That is not really true. The bacteria that cause Lyme disease have been making people sick for a long time. But Lyme disease was not identified and named until 1975. Before that, the symptoms were confused with other illnesses. People who had Lyme disease did not get the right kind of treatment and often kept getting sicker.

This book will explain how people get Lyme disease. It will tell you the symptoms of Lyme disease and how it is treated in case you do get it. You will learn what ticks look like and where they live. Most importantly, this book will help you protect yourself so that you do not get Lyme disease.

Lyme disease is not new. The bacteria and the infection have been around for a very long time. Scientists in Europe first knew and wrote about a disease like Lyme disease in 1883. In that year, a German doctor named Alfred Buchwald wrote about a rash that looked like the bull's-eye on a target, which was similar to the "bull's-eye rash" common with Lyme disease. During these early years, though, a link was not made between the rash and more severe symptoms. Even when doctors saw that patients with bull's-eye rashes also had joint pain or severe headaches, the doctors still did not know the cause.

A Mysterious Disease

Before the 1970s, people in the United States suffered from Lyme disease, but neither they nor their doctors knew it. Doctors had not identified the disease or the bacteria that cause it. Often, people who really had Lyme disease were diagnosed with other illnesses, such as the flu or multiple sclerosis. Sometimes they were told that their symptoms were psychosomatic. That means that doctors thought the patients were not really sick but were imagining their symptoms.

That is what some doctors told Polly Murray. They said she was imagining that she was sick and that it was all in her head. But Polly knew that they were wrong. Polly lived in Lyme, Connecticut. She had been sick on and off for more than ten years. Her head and neck ached constantly. A rash appeared on her hands, disappeared, then appeared again. She had terrible pain in her joints and sometimes had to keep her arm in a sling. For more than ten years, she was tested for many diseases, but doctors never could find the cause of her symptoms.

In the summer of 1975, Polly and her whole family were very sick. Her husband had trouble talking because he had laryngitis. He had to walk with crutches because of knee pain. Her sons seemed to have juvenile rheumatoid arthritis, a disease that causes children to have stiff and painful swollen joints. One son also had vision problems. At one point, her daughter's tongue swelled so much that she almost missed her high school graduation. They also had strange rashes. At times, their symptoms would seem to be cured, but they kept coming back. Even their dog was sick.

Polly knew something was terribly wrong, but the doctors she took her family to could not help her. She thought perhaps the drinking water in her home had been polluted and was making her family sick. But when she tested the water, it was fine.

The Mystery Is Uncovered

Polly began talking to her neighbors. She found that many of them had the same kinds of problems. Finally, in October of 1975, she called the Connecticut Health Department. The people she spoke to there suggested that she talk to Dr. Allen Steere, a doctor at Yale University. Dr. Steere was interested in studying arthritis. Arthritis was not considered to be a contagious disease—most doctors believed that you could not "catch" arthritis from someone who already has it. But Dr. Steere thought it might be possible to catch it. To prove whether his idea was true, he would need to find a group of people who lived near each other and had arthritis.

Dr. Steere and other doctors who worked with him began seeing and talking to people in Lyme, Connecticut, who had stiff and swollen joints. By May 1976, they had found thirty-nine children and twelve adults who lived in or near Lyme and had the symptoms of arthritis. Dr. Steere believed that he had found a new kind of arthritis, which he named "Lyme arthritis," after the town where the sufferers lived. Later, though, doctors came to understand that the disease affecting Polly, her family, and others in the town was different from arthritis. This new disease had many other symptoms, including rashes, headaches, vision trouble, and stomach problems. The name of the disease was changed to Lyme disease.

Recognizing the disease was an important step, but scientists and doctors still had a long way to go. They did not know what caused Lyme disease or how to treat it. Soon Dr. Steere began to suspect that tick bites had something to do with the disease. The people he had examined all had been bitten by ticks before they developed symptoms. But no one was sure which kind of

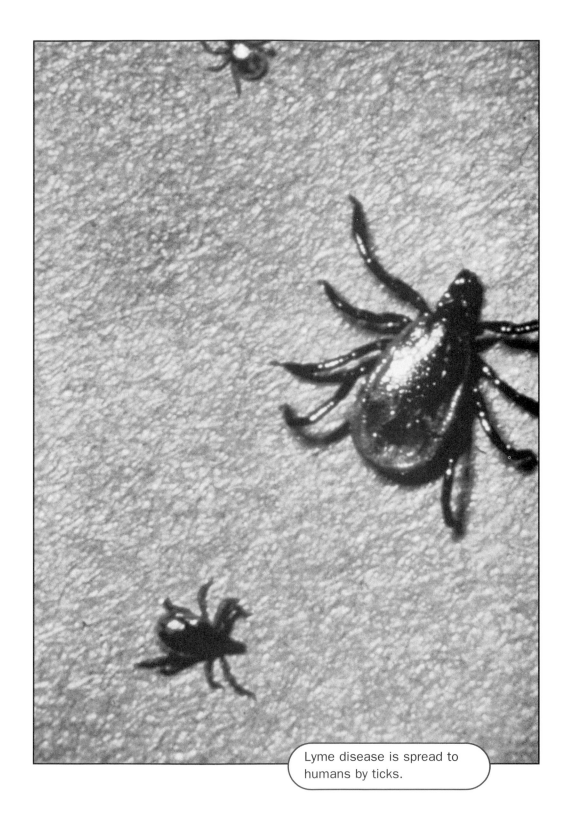

Lyme disease is spread to humans by ticks.

tick carried the disease or what caused the disease in ticks. Finally, in 1979, Dr. Andrew Spielman showed that the deer tick (also called the black-legged tick) carries a type of bacteria that causes Lyme disease. When deer ticks bite people, they pass this bacteria on to them.

Now scientists knew how people got Lyme disease. Doctors still had questions, however. What kind of bacteria causes the infection? How does the infection get from the tick to a human? Without knowing the answers to these questions, they could not begin to treat the disease.

At the Rocky Mountain Laboratories, part of the National Institutes of Health, in Montana, Dr. Willy Burgdorfer had been studying a different disease called Rocky Mountain spotted fever. This disease is also caused by ticks. Dr. Burgdorfer and his colleagues looked at bacteria carried by different types of ticks, including the tiny, black-legged deer tick. They discovered that the deer tick did not carry Rocky Mountain spotted fever. But they did find a strange, unfamiliar kind of spirochete (a type of bacteria) in the deer ticks that they studied. They checked blood samples taken from Lyme disease patients and found that the blood samples held the same kind of spirochete. They knew then that these spirochetes must be the cause of Lyme disease. In 1984, the bacteria were given the scientific name *Borrelia burgdorferi,* after Dr. Burgdorfer.

Doctors continued to study Lyme disease. Nowadays they know a lot more about this disease and how to treat it. They know that taking an antibiotic—a type of substance that destroys bacteria—will probably cure most people who get treatment right away. But some people suffered from Lyme disease before doctors knew what it was or how to treat it. Antibiotics do not seem to work well for these people, and some of them still have very severe health problems today. In addition, for a variety of reasons, antibiotics have not helped some people who developed Lyme disease after doctors began to understand it.

Chapter Two

Understanding Lyme Disease

Ticks, mice, and deer carry the Lyme disease bacteria called *Borrelia burgdorferi*. This thin, spiral kind of bacteria is called a spirochete. The bacteria do not make mice and deer sick. But when a tick bites a mouse or deer that carries the bacteria in its blood, the tick gets the bacteria, too. If you are bitten by this infected tick, you will also get the bacteria. And you will very likely get sick.

When an infected tick bites you, it sends the bacteria into your bloodstream. If it is left untreated, the bacteria can travel all over your body. Most often the bacteria travel to your joints and nervous system.

What Is Lyme Disease Like?

Billy West spent the first week of his summer vacation visiting his grandparents in Connecticut. A few days after he got home to New York City, he was combing his hair and noticed a strange red rash on his neck. He showed the rash to his mom.

"I've never seen anything like that," she said. "Is it itchy?"

"No," Billy said, "It doesn't hurt, either. But it's really weird. It looks like rings."

"Does anything else hurt?" she asked.

"Yes, I have a headache," Billy said.

Billy's mom took his temperature. It was about 100 degrees.

"I think we'd better call the doctor and get to the bottom of this," Billy's mom said.

Stage I: Erythema Migrans

The first symptom of Lyme disease that you see is often (but not always) a spreading skin rash called *erythema migrans,* or EM. *Erythema migrans* means "wandering redness." You can tell that you have an EM rash in these ways:

1. It usually is lighter in the center where the tick bit you. Around the bite spot you will find darker red rings. The rash starts small. Then, as time goes on, it spreads outward from the bite. These rings have given the rash its nickname, the bull's-eye rash. Sometimes, though, the whole rash is solid red.

2. Most often, the rash shows up within one to two weeks after you have been bitten. It could appear as soon as three days or as late as thirty days after you have been bitten. When you see the rash, the Lyme disease bacteria have already been sent into your bloodstream. In fact, researchers have found that the Lyme bacteria may already have reached the fluid around your spinal cord at this time.

3. The rash can be from two to twenty-four inches across. The most common size is five to six inches across. The rash usually lasts for about three to five weeks.

4. An EM rash is not painful or itchy. Sometimes it may feel warm to the touch.

On light-skinned people, an EM rash is easy to see. On people with dark or tanned skin, the rash may look like a bruise. Along with the rash, you may have a slight fever, a mild headache, and general achiness. These early symptoms, usually called Stage I, are very much like the flu. Often, people who do not see a rash will think that their aches and fever are caused by the flu. They may not even go to the doctor, because the symptoms are so mild. In these cases, treatment may not start until the Lyme disease bacteria have spread. As a result, the infection may advance to Stage II and cause more serious problems.

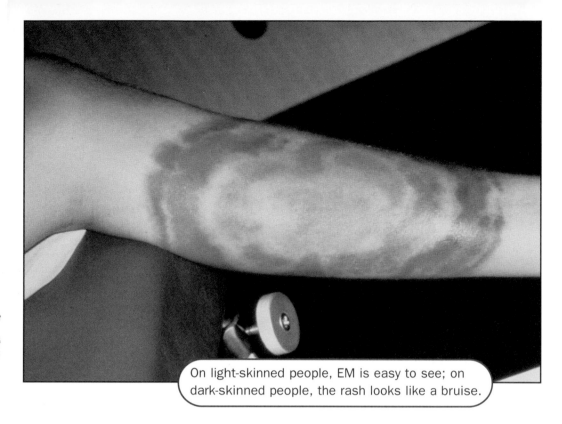

On light-skinned people, EM is easy to see; on dark-skinned people, the rash looks like a bruise.

Stage II: Disseminated Lyme Disease

Stage II Lyme disease is sometimes called disseminated Lyme disease. This means that the Lyme disease has spread to several parts of your body.

One evening, Samantha Armstrong limped into the living room and told her parents, Allison and Rob, that her knee hurt. "Did you twist it when you were playing softball today?" Rob asked.

"I'm not sure," answered Samantha. "I did slide into second base. Maybe I hurt my knee then."

"Why don't we wait and see how it feels in the morning?" suggested Allison.

When Samantha went to bed, her knee still hurt. By morning, it was much worse. "Mom,

Dad," she called. "My knee is really swollen. I don't think I can walk!"

Allison and Rob tried to help Samantha stand, but she could not put any weight on her knee. They called the doctor, who told them to come to his office right away. Rob had to carry Samantha to the car.

In children, the most common symptom of Stage II Lyme disease is painful, swollen joints, a kind of arthritis. According to a study in the *Journal of Pediatrics*, in over 90 percent of the time, children's knees are affected by this Lyme arthritis.

Lyme arthritis can come on very quickly. In twenty-four hours, you may go from feeling fine to being unable to walk. If you have not seen the EM rash, you may assume that you do not have Lyme disease and instead find yourself trying to think of a recent time when you might have hurt your knee. "Did I bruise my knee when I fell off my bike?" "Did I twist my knee playing basketball?" These questions may seem like logical ones to ask, but focusing on them could delay the proper treatment.

By the time Samantha, Rob, and Allison got to the doctor's office, they were very worried. Dr. Carey asked them if Samantha had hurt her knee, and they told him about the softball game. Then Dr. Carey asked them some questions that they weren't expecting.

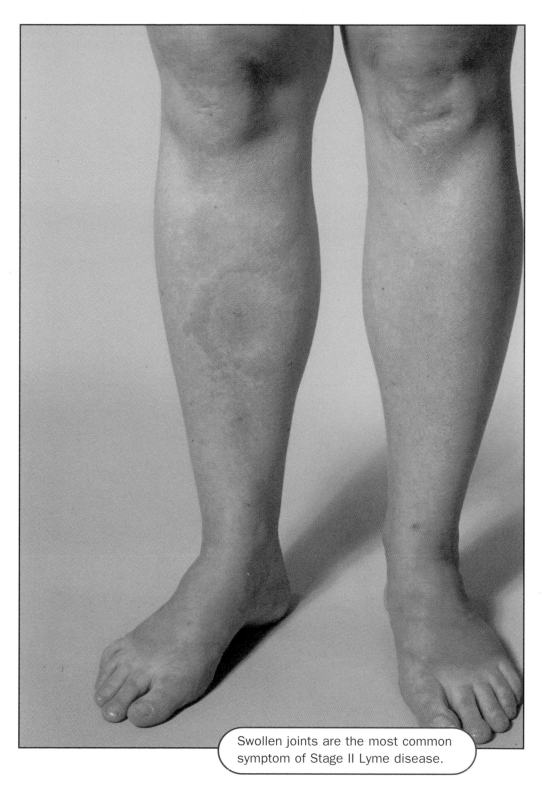

Swollen joints are the most common symptom of Stage II Lyme disease.

"Samantha, do you spend a lot of time outside?"

"I guess so," Samantha answered. "I have soft-ball practice every day after school and games on the weekends."

"When you're waiting for your turn at bat, do you sit on the grass?"

"Well, yes," she said. "During the games, we always sit on the bench. But at practice sometimes we sit on the ground. It's cooler on the grass under the trees."

"Do you wear shorts to practice?" asked Dr. Carey.

"Yes, usually."

"I don't think that your swollen knee is caused by an injury," said Dr. Carey. "I think that you have Lyme disease. It's caused by a bite from a tick that is infected with Lyme bacteria. Since you spend a lot of time sitting on the ground, it is very possible a tick could have bitten you. Do you remember finding a tick?"

"She did have a tick, but we pulled it off right away," said Allison. "And she never had a bull's-eye rash. Don't you have to have that rash to have Lyme disease?"

"Not everyone gets the rash," said Dr. Carey. "That's one of the reasons that Lyme disease can be so hard to diagnose. With the rash, it's pretty easy. But people who don't get the rash can have the Lyme bacteria in their bodies for months before they get any Lyme disease symptoms. They

may feel achy or have a headache, but they usually just think that they have the flu."

"What should we do now? Will she be okay?" asked Rob.

"She should be fine. We'll take her to the hospital, where they can do some tests to be sure we're right. They will also give her some strong antibiotics. She'll take more antibiotics at home for a while. Most likely, she'll be fine."

Lyme disease can also affect your nervous system. You may have a stiff neck or very bad headaches. The muscles in your face may become paralyzed, making one side of your face look droopy. This condition is called Bell's palsy. These symptoms can occur several weeks, months, or even years after an untreated infection from a tick bite.

Although these symptoms are the most common, people with Lyme disease, especially adults, can have many other symptoms. Lyme disease has been called "the great imitator" because it can seem to be so many other diseases. This can make it hard for doctors to know for sure that you have Lyme disease. People with Stage II Lyme disease can also have these symptoms:

- The same flulike symptoms, including severe headache, nausea, lack of energy, and vomiting, may show up, go away, then come back several times.

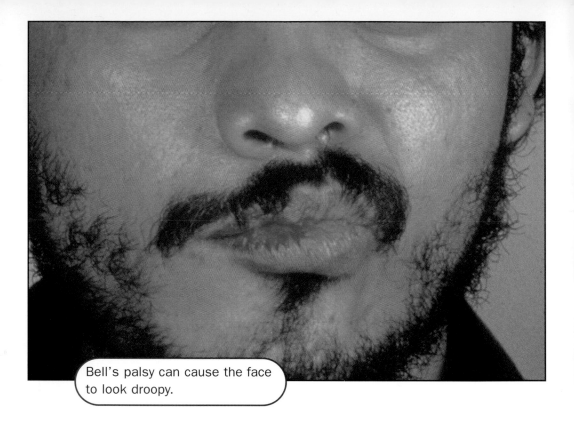

Bell's palsy can cause the face to look droopy.

- You may lose your appetite and/or have diarrhea.

- You may feel confused or forgetful.

- You may be irritable and get annoyed very easily.

- You may be very sensitive to light, so that all but the dimmest light is painful to your eyes.

- You may lose some part of your vision.

- You may lose your ability to smell. Or the opposite could happen and odors may seem very strong.

- You may lose part of your hearing or have a ringing in your ears.

- Your fingers and toes may feel numb or tingly.

- You may find it hard to concentrate or you may feel dizzy at times.

- You may lose coordination and feel clumsy.

- You may have an irregular heartbeat, which may be caused by the bacteria's damage to your heart.

- You may find it hard to breathe.

Other major organs that may be affected during Stage II Lyme disease include your liver, lungs, intestines, spleen, bladder, and kidneys. Fortunately, these symptoms are rare.

Samantha and her parents arrived at the hospital and were sent to the emergency room. They sat in the waiting room until their name was called. Then they were led to an examining room.

"Hello, Samantha. I'm Dr. Kelly," said a tall blond woman. "I'm going to examine you and take some tests to find out what is causing your knee pain. Dr. Monroe is going to help me." Dr. Monroe stood behind Dr. Kelly. Samantha thought he looked very young.

"I'm going to need to take some blood from your arm, Samantha. It may hurt a bit, but I'll do my best to be very careful," said Dr. Kelly. "Mrs. Armstrong, you might want to hold Samantha's hand until I'm finished."

Dr. Kelly used a needle to take some blood from Samantha's arm. When she was finished, she said, "I also need to take some of the fluid from around your knee. The fluid is what makes your knee look swollen. Testing that fluid will help us be sure that you do not have an infection caused by an injury. That will help us confirm that you have Lyme disease."

Doctors often find it hard to know for sure when you have Lyme disease because other conditions or infections can also cause these symptoms. This can work against you in two ways. First, the doctor may start treatment for another illness that he or she thinks is the cause of your symptoms. In this case, the Lyme disease may not be treated properly and it could get worse. On the other hand, a doctor may start treatment for Lyme disease when the symptoms were really caused by another disease, such as multiple sclerosis. You may get treatment that you do not need for Lyme disease while the true problem is left untreated.

Stage III: Chronic Lyme Disease

Stage III, or chronic (constant and ongoing) Lyme disease, is the most dangerous form. Symptoms that seem to have disappeared come back and get worse. Chronic arthritis, especially of the knees, sets in. Pain and swelling can make walking nearly impossible. The pain and stiffness may last for a few days or weeks, then seem to heal. But the symptoms return, over and over. In the chronic stage, many of the Stage II symptoms return again and again and keep getting worse.

Doctors, however, do not agree about what is really happening during this stage of the disease. Dr. Allen Steere, the doctor who first worked on Lyme disease in 1975, now thinks that many people who think that they have Lyme disease do not really have it. In an article published in the *Journal of the American Medical Association* in 1993, Dr. Steere said that Lyme disease is diagnosed too often. The doctors give people medicine that may not help them if they do not really have Lyme disease. He believes that the symptoms that keep coming back are caused by a condition he calls "post-Lyme syndrome." He thinks that the damage to the body may first have been caused by Lyme disease. But he thinks that "post-Lyme syndrome" is really a new disease. The important difference is in the treatment. Dr. Steere believes that giving people antibiotics for a very long time is not the best solution for chronic Lyme disease.

This has caused some problems for people whose doctors disagree with Dr. Steere. These doctors are still telling their patients to take antibiotics for a long time to help fight their Lyme disease. Dr. Steere said that this treatment will not work, so some insurance companies have said that they will not pay for it.

Chapter Three

Diagnosing and Treating Lyme Disease

Dr. Kelly met with Samantha and her parents. "I have your test results, Samantha," she said. "As we thought, you have Lyme disease. The infection has already spread to your joints. So we will need to give you antibiotics intravenously for two days. You will need to stay overnight in the hospital. But after the antibiotics begin working, you can go home. You'll take pills after you're home until the infection is gone."

"May I stay here with her overnight?" asked Allison.

"Of course," said Dr. Kelly. "And don't worry. Samantha should be fine."

Lyme disease can sometimes be hard to diagnose. If you do not get the EM rash, you may think that your early symptoms are caused by some other, more common

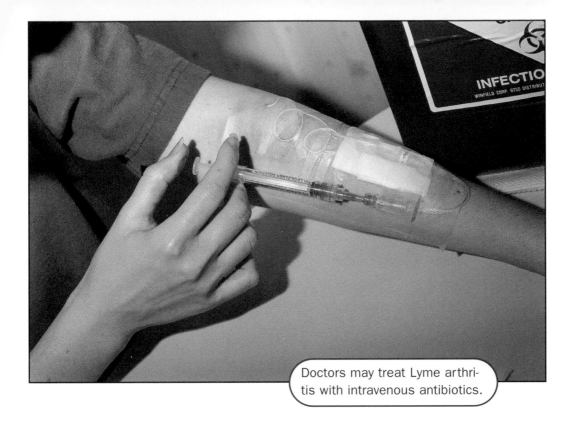

Doctors may treat Lyme arthritis with intravenous antibiotics.

illness, such as the flu. Stage II and III Lyme disease can be mistaken for other serious conditions. The joint pain of Lyme arthritis can be mistaken for rheumatoid arthritis. Symptoms that affect the brain and nervous system are sometimes confused with multiple sclerosis.

According to the Centers for Disease Control (CDC), when your doctor checks your physical symptoms, he or she should also ask you some important questions. These questions could help to find out if a tick bit you:

- Do you live in, or were you visiting, an area where deer ticks are common?

- Have you recently spent time outdoors, especially in wooded areas or places with tall grass?

• Do you like to go hiking, fishing, or hunting?

• How often do you spend time outside?

• Do you remember finding a tick on your body?

It is important to answer as completely as possible. Remember that you could have been bitten by a tick weeks, or even months, before the doctor asks these questions. You will need to think very carefully to help your doctor find out if you have Lyme disease.

There are also blood tests to help doctors diagnose Lyme disease. These tests, though, are not always correct, especially in the first stage of Lyme disease. Up to a month after an infected tick bites you, the tests may not show a positive result, even though you are infected. This is because the test looks for antibodies, the cells that your body makes to fight off the disease. Your body may not have made enough antibodies yet for Lyme disease. Some tests cannot tell the difference between Lyme antibodies and antibodies for other diseases. On the other hand, you may test positive for Lyme disease when your symptoms are really caused by something else. To make things even more complicated, people who have gotten a Lyme disease vaccination to protect themselves against the disease will also test positive.

Tests for finding out if you have Stage II and III Lyme disease are much more certain. However, they still are not 100 percent right all the time. According to

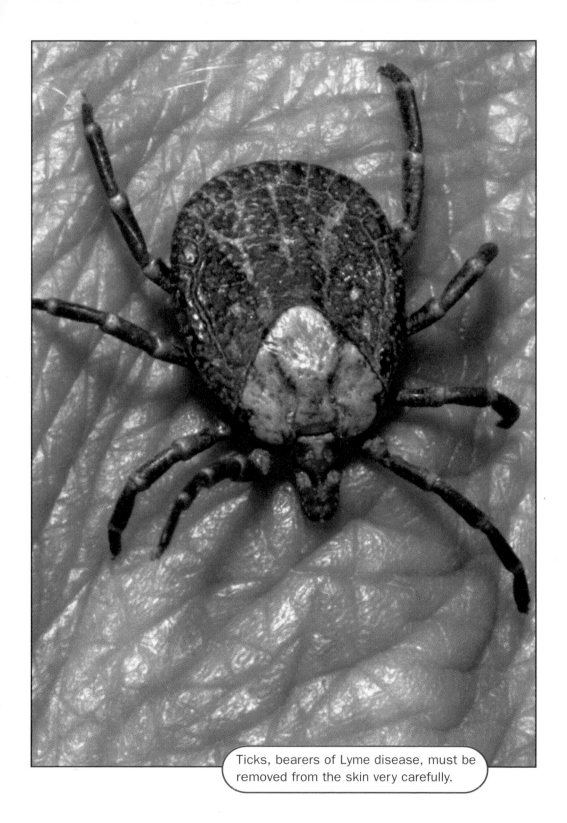

Ticks, bearers of Lyme disease, must be removed from the skin very carefully.

the Lyme Disease Foundation, no test can truly rule out Lyme disease. Scientists are still working to find better tests that will give a correct result more often.

What Are the Treatments?

Mrs. West took Billy to see Dr. Wesley the day after Billy showed her the red rash on his neck.

"Let's see that rash, Billy," said Dr. Wesley. Billy pulled his shirt collar away from his neck. "That looks like the EM rash, which is a symptom of Lyme disease. Have you been walking in the woods recently?"

"Yes, I was visiting my grandparents in Connecticut," said Billy. "I love to take their golden retriever running in the woods."

"Well, Lyme disease is caused by a tick bite, and ticks live in the woods," Dr. Wesley said. "You probably would not find many ticks in the city, but there are lots of them in the woods in Connecticut. I'll give your mom a prescription for an antibiotic. That's the kind of medicine that fights Lyme disease. You can pick it up at the drugstore on the way home. Since you found your rash right away, the medicine should work quickly. But if you feel any pain in your knees or if they look swollen, call me right away."

"Okay, Dr. Wesley," said Billy. "Thanks."

According to the American Lyme Disease Foundation, if you begin treatment within three weeks of the day

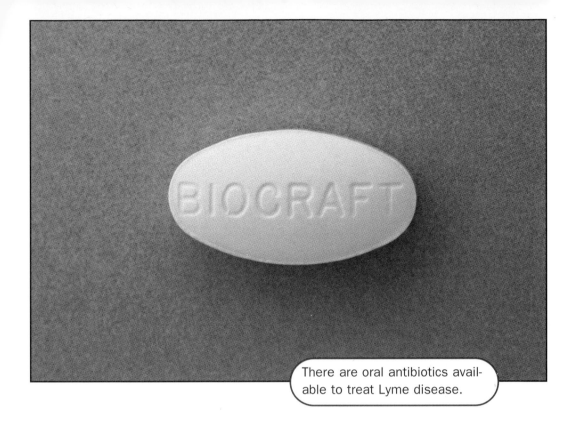

There are oral antibiotics available to treat Lyme disease.

you were infected, Lyme disease is almost always easily cured. Most likely, your doctor will give you antibiotics to take. Sometimes Lyme arthritis is treated by taking oral antibiotics for thirty days. These antibiotics may be in pill or liquid form. Other doctors may treat Lyme arthritis with intravenous antibiotics. Intravenous means that the medicine is sent directly into your bloodstream through a tube attached to a needle. To get intravenous antibiotics, you will need to stay in the hospital for a day or two. If the disease has affected your heart or nervous system, you will be given intravenous antibiotics as soon as your doctor has diagnosed you.

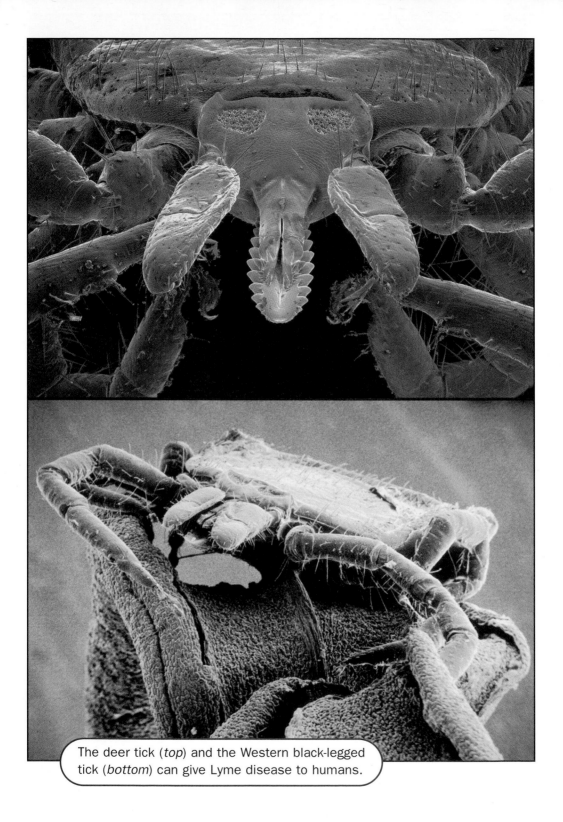

The deer tick (*top*) and the Western black-legged tick (*bottom*) can give Lyme disease to humans.

Chapter Four

Ticks

What are ticks? If your answer is "creepy bugs that serve no useful purpose," many people, including Karen Vanderhoof-Forschner, founder of the Lyme Disease Foundation, would agree with you. Ticks are arachnids, a group of animals that also includes spiders. Ticks are not insects. Ticks have three body sections, whereas insects have two, and adult ticks have eight legs, unlike insects, which have six. Ticks do not have wings or antennae, as insects do.

Ticks are parasites. They live off the blood of a person or another animal, called the host. Parasites cannot survive on their own and depend on their host for food and to reproduce. In other word, ticks are a pain!

There are more than 850 species, or kinds, of ticks in the world. In North America, five kinds of ticks can give disease to humans. The black-legged tick, sometimes called the deer or bear tick, carries Lyme disease bacteria from eastern North America through the Midwest. Along the Pacific Coast and in the northwestern United States, the disease is carried by the Western black-legged tick. If you live in the Northeast, you may be familiar with the dog tick. As its name suggests, this tick often lives on dogs. Dog ticks are larger than deer ticks, and they do not carry Lyme disease.

The Life Cycle of a Tick

The life cycle of a tick lasts two years and has four stages. In each stage, the tick molts, or sheds, its old skeleton and grows a new one to fit its new body shape. The four phases are:

1. **Egg**. In the fall and early spring, adult ticks mate on the bodies of large animals such as white-tailed deer. The female needs to feed off a host in order for her to produce her eggs. She then drops off from the deer to lay the eggs on the ground. The eggs hatch into larvae by summer.

2. **Larvae**. Sometimes called seed ticks, larvae have six legs and are very tiny. They feed for about two days on mice and other small mammals and birds during the summer and into early fall. That one meal will be enough to last them until the

next spring, when they will feed and molt into nymphs.

3. **Nymph**. At this stage, the tick has all eight of its legs. It is now the size of a poppy seed, or the period at the end of this sentence. Nymphs feed for about four days in the late spring and summer and molt into adults in the fall. You are most likely to get Lyme disease from nymphs because they are the most active in spring and summer, and you probably spend the most time outside when the weather is warm. Nymphs are also very hard to see because they are so tiny.

4. **Adult.** In this final stage, the tick is the size of a sesame seed. When the female feeds, it swells, or becomes engorged, until it is about the size of a pea.

Ticks can become infected with Lyme disease bacteria during the last three stages. They carry the bacteria with them when they molt, infecting more mice, deer, and people when they feed on them.

If ticks could choose their hosts, they would not choose you. They much prefer deer or mice. But they will take advantage of any chance to hitch a ride for a meal. If the opportunity arises, ticks will feed on raccoons, chipmunks, dogs, cats, or cattle. In fact, scientists

it down the toilet. Do not squash the tick, especially if it has become swelled, because you may release infected blood. Be sure to wash your hands after removing the tick.

Some people may suggest that you cover the tick with petroleum jelly to smother it. But ticks need very little oxygen to live, and by the time an infected tick runs out of air, you will be infected, too. Another suggestion is to hold a hot match against the tick to make it release its hold and back out. Remember, ticks are tiny! You are much more likely to burn yourself than to make a tick move. Using tweezers to carefully pull out the tick is the best way to remove it.

Over the next several days, Michael and his mom often checked the spot where they had removed the tick. Michael did not get a rash of any kind, and he felt fine. "I don't think you have Lyme disease," his mother said. "Just be sure to let me know if your knees hurt. And next time, before you go out in the woods, think about ticks and wear different clothes."

Chapter Five | Protection Against Lyme Disease

M*ichael was heading out to meet Jason and Matt at their favorite spot in the woods. "Wait a minute," said his mother. "You can't go out in the woods in shorts and sandals. Remember the tick? Please change into long pants and a long-sleeved shirt. Wear socks and sneakers."*

"Oh, Mom, I don't want to do that," said Michael. "I'll be too hot."

"Well, you have to," said his mother. "It will be cool in the woods, and you'll be fine. Besides, it's better than taking the chance of getting Lyme disease."

The best way to protect yourself from Lyme disease is to stay out of the woods. Avoid areas with tall grass. Never sit on the grass. Walk around piles of dead leaves. It is safest to stay indoors. But most of us would rather not spend a sunny summer day gazing out the window. Chances are, you enjoy hiking, gardening, hunting, fishing, or other outdoor activities. Especially if you live or take vacations in places where deer ticks are found, the American Lyme Disease Foundation suggests that you follow this advice:

1. Wear light-colored clothing made with a tight weave. You will be able to spot ticks more easily and they will have trouble getting to your skin.

2. Always wear enclosed shoes or boots. Save your sandals for the beach.

3. Wear long pants tucked into your socks and long-sleeved shirts tucked into your pants.

4. Before you head into the woods, you may want to spray your clothes with insect repellent containing the insecticide DEET. Another insect repellent, permethrin, also works against ticks. Spray permethrin on your clothes before you put them on, then let them dry for at least two hours before you wear them. Karen Vanderhoof-Forschner of the Lyme Disease Foundation recommends Avon's Skin-So-Soft Bug Guard Mosquito Repellent.

5. Wear a hat. Keep long hair pulled back so that it does not brush against bushes or tall grass.

6. When gardening, pruning, or picking up dead leaves, wear light-colored gloves and check them frequently for ticks.

7. Avoid sitting on the ground or on stone walls where ticks may hide. If you go to an outdoor concert, picnic, or other event where you must sit on the ground, use a blanket that has been sprayed with an insect repellent like the ones recommended in step 4.

8. When hiking, stay on cleared, well-traveled paths whenever possible.

9. While you are out in the woods or working in your garden, check yourself and others for ticks every three or four hours. Do not give them a chance to climb under your clothes.

10. When you get home from your outdoor activities, change your clothes right away. It's best to remove your outer layer of clothes away from the living area of your house—for example, in the basement or garage. Check the clothes for ticks and wash them as soon as possible.

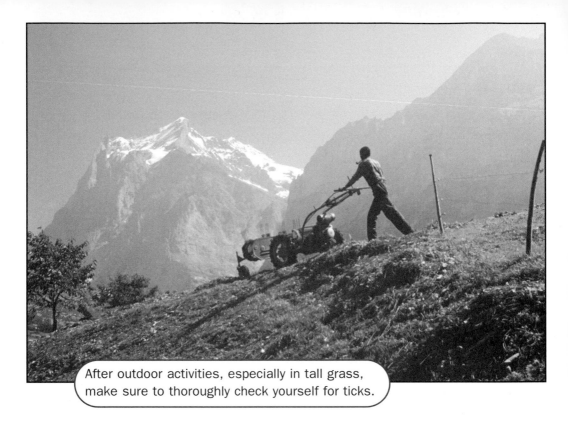

After outdoor activities, especially in tall grass, make sure to thoroughly check yourself for ticks.

11. Take a shower and wash your hair, checking your entire body for ticks. They like to crawl into places where it will be hard to find them. Look behind your knees, in your navel, behind your ears, at the back of your neck, in your armpits—everywhere! Pay special attention to areas where underwear elastic, waistbands from pants, and shirt collars touch your skin. Use a hand-held mirror to check hard-to-see places.

In addition to protecting your body, you can also make it harder for ticks to live around your house. If you have a lawn, keep it mowed. Ticks like tall, moist, grassy areas. Clear brush and leaf litter away from the house, garden, or stone walls. If you have a fireplace, be sure to stack woodpiles neatly in a dry location. Mice often make nests in woodpiles.

If you have a bird feeder, keep the ground under it clean so you do not attract mice and chipmunks. A fence can keep deer, and the ticks that they carry, away from your home.

"We need to do everything we can to make sure none of us get Lyme disease again," said Samantha's dad, Rob. "Let's clean up our yard to keep ticks as far away from us as we can."

"Good idea," said Allison, Samantha's mom. "We can start by cutting back that high grass along the fence."

"We can rake up all the dead leaves, too," said Samantha. "They blow under the bushes and get stuck there. Ticks love to hide in damp, cool places like that."

"If we keep the yard clean, ticks will have a harder time living there," said Rob. "And we will be safer."

Where the Ticks Are

Knowing where you are most likely to find infected ticks will help you to protect yourself from the disease. According to the Centers for Disease Control,

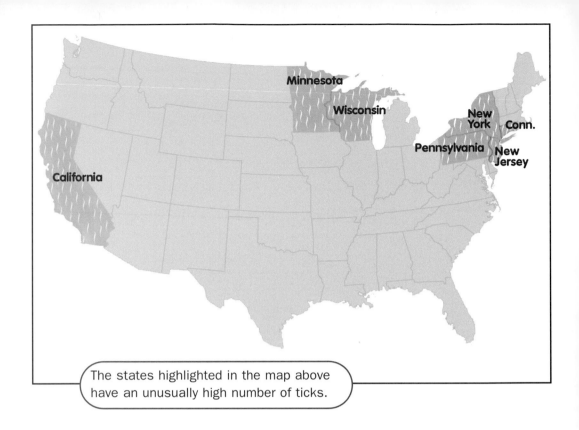

The states highlighted in the map above have an unusually high number of ticks.

you are most likely to get Lyme disease in the Northeastern United States. New York, New Jersey, Pennsylvania, and Connecticut all reported more than 2,000 cases in 1997. Other high incidence states include California, Minnesota and Wisconsin. Connecticut's incidence rate (the number of cases per 100,000 people) of 70.23 is more than double nearly every other state's. Montana is the only state in the country with no cases reported to the CDC.

You should keep in mind, however, that these numbers show only cases that were reported to the CDC. In Connecticut, doctors know what the symptoms of Lyme disease look like and are more likely to report it. Because the symptoms can seem to be the same as those of other illnesses, many cases of Lyme disease may never be reported. This is especially true in states where there are not many cases. Doctors sometimes do not recognize it. Other times, doctors may confuse a patient's symptoms and diagnose Lyme disease when the symptoms are actually caused by another kind of infection.

You do not need to live in a high-risk area to be infected. Whether you plan to vacation in the woods of Wisconsin or on the beaches of Cape Cod, Massachusetts, be careful. Not only can you become infected while on vacation, you can bring ticks home with you on your clothing or camping gear. Also, some researchers believe that ticks can hitch a ride on migrating birds and come to you wherever you live.

You can be bitten at any time of the year, but the peak season is April to September in the Northeast and November to April on the West Coast.

In Canada, Lyme disease has been diagnosed in Alberta, New Brunswick, Quebec, Ontario, Manitoba, Saskatchewan, and British Columbia. It occurs throughout Europe, all over Russia and the surrounding countries, and in parts of Africa, Australia, China, and Japan.

A Tick's Home

Ticks like shady, moist areas. They are most often found near the ground, in dead leaves, or on low weeds.

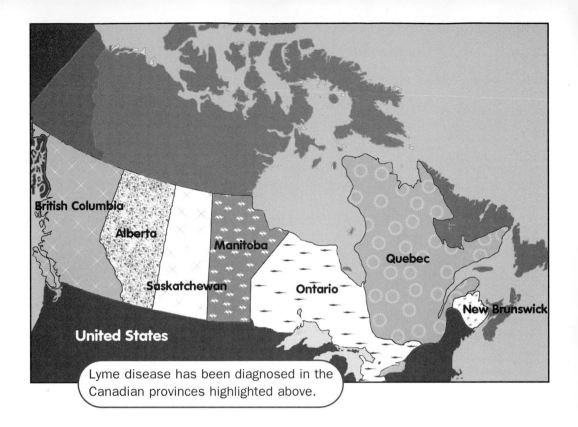

Lyme disease has been diagnosed in the Canadian provinces highlighted above.

They can also cling to tall grass and shrubs, up to three feet from the ground. But they cannot fly, and they will not jump on to you from a higher perch. A tick must be able to touch you. From its perch on a leaf or twig, the tick waves its front legs in the air, behavior that scientists call "questing." It uses scent to tell it that a host is nearby. It can also find a host by sensing body heat. Claws and sticky pads at the tips of its legs help it to latch onto the host. Most likely, after reaching your skin, the tick will crawl upward to a warmer, more hidden spot, such as the back of your knee or your armpit.

There are more cases of Lyme disease in the Northeast because large numbers of deer and white-footed mice live there. Ticks need deer and mice to survive and reproduce. Mice and deer carry the bacteria and infected ticks, but do not get sick.

Protecting Yourself

Lyme disease can be very dangerous. You can lessen the danger by protecting yourself when you are outside in a place where ticks live. Wear long-sleeved shirts, long pants, socks, and closed shoes when hiking or playing in the woods or in tall grass. Check yourself for ticks when you come inside. If you see a spreading red EM rash on your skin, tell your parents and go to the doctor right away. Start treatment as soon as you can.

You may be infected with Lyme disease even if you have never had the EM rash. Swollen joints (especially knees), headache, and achiness are symptoms of disseminated Lyme disease. Disseminated Lyme disease can lead to more serious symptoms. If you live in an area where deer ticks are found, it is smart to understand the symptoms of Lyme disease. Most importantly, protect yourself and your pets from tick bites.

Protecting Your Pets

Dogs and cats can get Lyme disease, too. First and most importantly, remember that you are your pet's best defense against Lyme disease. Your dog or cat cannot protect itself. There are now several products that you can get from your veterinarian that will repel ticks.

Talk to your vet and find out what he or she suggests. Your vet can also tell you about the anti-Lyme vaccine for dogs. Scientists are still working on new treatments. Again, your vet can give you the most up-to-date information.

For several reasons, your dog is much more likely to become infected with Lyme disease than you are. Dogs need to spend time out-of-doors. Unleashed dogs pay no attention to paths, choosing instead to follow their noses, even if they end up crashing through the underbrush. Ticks are hard to see against a dog's fur, especially when it is a dark color.

When should you worry that your dog is infected? Sometimes it is hard to tell. Your dog may seem to have less energy than usual and sleep more of the time. She may have a fever or eat less. She may also have stiff, painful joints. If you know that your dog has not had any injury but seems to be having a hard time walking, you should probably ask your vet to test her for Lyme disease. If you find the infection early and give your dog antibiotics, she should be fine in a short time.

Cats seem to get Lyme disease less often than dogs. This could be because cats groom themselves often. A tick may be licked away before it has a chance to bite. Still, if you have an outdoor cat and live in an area where deer ticks are common, there is a risk that it will be bitten by a tick and become infected with Lyme disease.

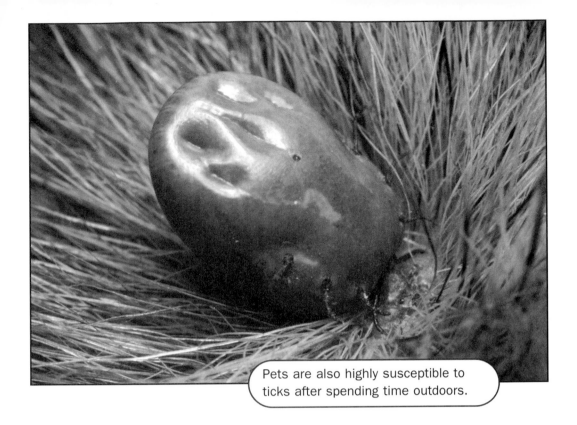

Pets are also highly susceptible to ticks after spending time outdoors.

Check your pet for ticks. If you find one stuck to your pet's skin, take it off with tweezers, just as you would remove it from yourself. Not only can your pet become infected, it can also bring ticks into the house, where they can drop off. Those ticks may choose you for their next meal!

Will a Vaccination Protect You?

On December 21, 1998, the United States Food and Drug Administration approved a Lyme disease vaccine. This first vaccine was not tested on children, so as of December 1999, it had not been approved for anyone younger than age fifteen.

According to the *New England Journal of Medicine,* the vaccine was tested on nearly 10,000 healthy people, ages fifteen to seventy, who live in places where Lyme disease is common. To get the highest level of protection, a person needs a series of three shots. The first two shots are given a month apart. They provide about 50 percent protection. A third shot, given eleven months later, increases protection to about 90 percent for people under age sixty-five.

If you are bitten by an infected tick, you can get Lyme disease even if you have already had it. According to the American Lyme Disease Foundation, the vaccine protects anyone who has already had Lyme disease in the same way it protects people who have never had it. But it will not protect against other diseases. The vaccine only sends antibodies against *Borrelia burgdorferi* bacteria. There is no scientific proof that you can get Lyme disease from the vaccine. However, after you have had the vaccine, you will test positive on at least one of the tests used to tell if you have the disease. In other words, after you have been vaccinated, this test will show that you have Lyme disease, even though you do not.

Researchers continue to test the vaccine to make it safe for children. They also hope to find a vaccine that will work using only one dose. The current vaccine may not be the best choice for most people, according to Dr. David Volkman, associate professor of medicine and pediatrics at the State University of New York at Stony Brook. The highest level of protection is not reached until a year after the first shot. Because the tests were done only during a two-year period, the vaccine has not been proven to work longer than that. So far, researchers do not know how long the effects of the vaccine will last. It may be necessary to get booster shots every year, beginning in the second year, to keep up the protection. Also, because the shots are so new, says Dr. Volkman, "We don't know the long-term effects of repeated doses of Lyme vaccine." Also, no one knows whether it is safe for people with chronic arthritis or undiagnosed Lyme disease.

Dr. Volkman also warns that being vaccinated may give you a false sense of security. "Even after you've had all three shots, you still need to take the normal precautions against Lyme disease, because the vaccine isn't 100 percent effective," he says.

Who should consider getting the Lyme disease vaccine? People who live in high-risk areas and spend a lot of time outdoors are the best candidates for the vaccine. If you live in Connecticut and your parents work in jobs that keep them outside, such as landscape or utility work, you may want to talk with them about the vaccine. Also, adults and teenagers in families who enjoy a lot of outdoor activities, such as hiking, camping, or hunting, may choose to be vaccinated. In other places, especially where deer ticks are not found very often, you may want to wait for

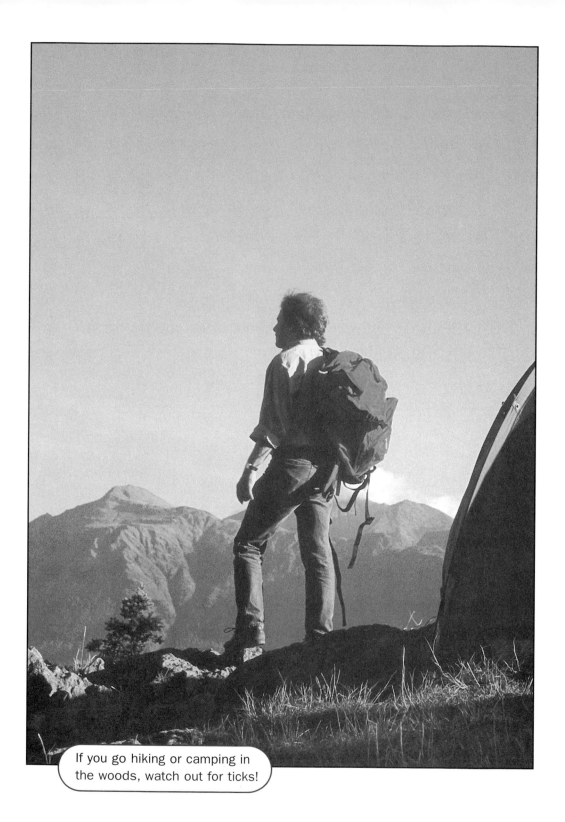

more research. People considering the vaccine should first talk to their doctor.

Remember that even those who are vaccinated are not 100 percent protected. You will still need to protect yourself in the same way you would if you had not received the vaccine. Lyme disease can be treated, but prevention is the most effective way to avoid the risks of this potentially serious disease.

Glossary

antibiotic A kind of medicine used to treat Lyme disease and other diseases that are caused by bacteria.

antibodies Cells that your body produces to fight off bacteria that cause disease.

arthritis Swollen and painful joints. Lyme arthritis is a symptom of Stage II, or disseminated, Lyme disease.

Bell's palsy A symptom of Stage II, or disseminated, Lyme disease. Muscles of the face droop on one side, making it difficult to smile.

Borrelia burgdorferi The bacteria that causes Lyme disease.

chronic Lyme disease Another name for Stage III Lyme disease. This is the most dangerous form of Lyme disease and can include heart and liver problems. Chronic Lyme disease is more common in adults and is relatively rare in young people.

contagious disease A disease that can be given to one person by someone who already has it.

disseminated Lyme disease The second stage of Lyme disease, in which the bacteria have spread through the body and are causing symptoms such as arthritis and Bell's palsy.

erythema migrans Often called the EM rash, this is the most common symptom of early Lyme disease. The rash is lighter in the center, around the bite wound. Red rings expand outward, giving this rash its nickname, the bull's-eye rash.

host The animal on whose blood ticks or other parasites feed.

intravenous Fed directly into the bloodstream, usually through a needle attached to a tube.

larva The second stage of a tick's life cycle, during which it has six legs and is very tiny.

molt To shed the hard outer skeleton. Ticks molt when changing life stages.

multiple sclerosis A disease that attacks the nervous system and is sometimes confused with Stage III Lyme disease.

nymph The third stage of a tick's life cycle, during which it is the size of a poppy seed and has eight legs. You are most likely to become infected with Lyme disease from a nymph.

parasite An animal or insect that lives off the blood of another animal, or host. It cannot find its own food and depends on the host animal for survival.

spirochete A spiral-shaped bacteria, such as the *Borrelia burgdorferi* bacteria that cause Lyme disease.

symptom A sign that you may have a disease. An EM rash, for example, is a symptom of Lyme disease.

Where to Go for Help

In the United States

American Lyme Disease Foundation
Mill Pond Offices
293 Route 100
Somers, NY 10589
(914) 277-6970
Web site: http://www.aldf.com

The Lyme Alliance
P.O. Box 454
Concord, MA 49237
Web site: http://www.lymealliance.org

Lyme Disease Foundation
One Financial Plaza

Hartford, CT 06103
(860) 525-2000
Web site: http://www.lyme.org

The Lyme Disease Network
43 Winton Road
East Brunswick, NJ 08816
Web site: http://www.lymenet.org

**National Institute for Arthritis and
    Musculoskeletal and Skin Diseases**
Lyme Disease Booklet NIH Publication No. 92-3193
NIAMS/NIH
1 AMS Circle
Bethesda, MD 20892
Web site: http://www.delphi.com/child/lyme.html

In Canada

Canadian Infectious Disease Society
2197 Promenade Riverside Drive, Suite 504
Pebb Building
Ottawa, ON K1H 7X3
(613) 260-3233
e-mail: cids@magma.ca
Web site: http://www.cids.medical.org

Laboratory Centre for Disease Control
Health Canada
Tunney's Pasture
Ottawa, ON K1A 0L2
Web site: http://www.hc-sc.gc.ca/hpb/lcdc/hp_eng.html

Web Sites

Health Canada
http://www.hc-sc.gc.ca/english

Lyme Disease
http://www.oldlymect.com/Lymedis.htm

Lyme Disease Information Resource
http://www.x-l.net/Lyme

National Center for Infectious Diseases—Lyme
Disease Brochure
http://www.cdc.gov/ncidod/diseases/lyme/lyme.htm

What Is Lyme Disease?
http://www.execpc.com/~jbehnke/page19.html

For Further Reading

Barbour, Alan G., M.D. *Lyme Disease: The Cause, The Cure, The Controversy*. Baltimore: Johns Hopkins Press, 1996.

Hoffman, Ronald L. *Lyme Disease.* New Canaan, CT: Keats Publishing, 1994.

Lang, Denise, with Joseph Territo. *Coping with Lyme Disease: A Practical Guide to Dealing with Diagnosis and Treatment*. New York: Henry Holt, 1997.

Mactire, Sean P. *Lyme Disease and Other Pest-Borne Illnesses*. Danbury, CT: Franklin Watts, 1991.

Murray, Polly. *The Widening Circle: A Lyme Disease Pioneer Tells Her Story*. New York: St. Martin's Press, 1996.

Rahn, Daniel W., M.D., and Janine Evans, M.D., eds. *Lyme Disease*. Philadelphia: American College of Physicians, 1998.

Silverstein, Alvin, Virginia Silverstein, and Robert Silverstein. *Lyme Disease, The Great Imitator: How to Prevent and Cure It*. Lebanon, NJ: AVSTAR Publishing, 1990.

Vanderhoof-Forschner, Karen. *Everything You Need to Know About Lyme Disease and Other Tick-Borne Disorders*. New York: John Wiley & Sons, 1997.

Veggeberg, Scott. *Lyme Disease*. Springfield, NJ: Enslow Publishing, 1998.

Index

About the Author

Karen Donnelly, a writer from Connecticut, has a master's degree in English literature from Southern Connecticut State University. She has written numerous books and newspaper and magazine articles for children and adults on such diverse topics as nature, architecture, careers, and health.

Photo Credits

Cover © Anthony Bannister, Gallo Images/CORBIS; p. 2 © Volker Steger/Peter Arnold, Inc.; p. 6 National Institute of Health/Science Photo Library/Custom Medical Stock Photo; pp. 11 and 17 © CDC/Peter Arnold, Inc.; p. 19 John Radcliffe Hospital/Science Photo Library/Custom Medical Stock Photo; p. 22 © Chat Childs/Peter Arnold, Inc.; p. 27 © Craig Newbauer/Peter Arnold, Inc.; p. 29 © Anthony Bannister, Gallo Images/CORBIS; p. 31 © Custom Medical Stock Photo; p. 32 (top) © David Scharf/Peter Arnold, Inc.; p. 32 (bottom) © Manfred Kage/Peter Arnold, Inc.; p. 37 © Mike Peres/Custom Medical Stock Photo; p. 42 © Kelly-Mooney Photography/CORBIS; pp. 44 and 46 © Magellan Geographix/CORBIS; p. 49 © Anthony Bannister, Gallo Images/CORBIS; p. 52 © Index Stock Photography, Inc.

Layout

Michael J. Caroleo